Let's Talk Sex & STDs
A Guide to Prepare Parents for "The Talk"

By: Dr. Katina Davis-Kennedy
EdD, MSN, ARNP, FNP-C

ISBN: 10:0996569421
ISBN: 13:978-0-9965694-2-2

Printed in the United States of America

For permission requests, write to the publisher, addressed "Attention: Permissions Coordinator," at the address below.

info@opportunepublishing.com
www.opportunepublishing.com

Disclaimer

Although the author and publisher have made every effort to ensure that the information in this book was correct at press time, the author and publisher do not assume and hereby disclaim any liability to any party for any loss, damage, or disruption caused by errors or omissions, whether such errors or omissions result from negligence, accident, or any other cause.

Call to press

If you are interested in booking this author for readings or other events, please use the contact information below.

Email:Katinadkennedy@gmail.com

Website: www.drkatinakennedy.com

Facebook: DrKatinaKennedy

Instagram:@Katinakennedynursepractitioner

YouTube: NurseK Kennedy

.

About the Author

Dr. Katina Davis-Kennedy resides from sunny Ft. Lauderdale, Florida. She has been in the nursing profession since 2003 and has continued to build such an adept career within the medical industry. Dr. Davis-Kennedy began her journey studying nursing at Florida A&M University, and then went on to complete her master's in nursing at Florida Atlantic University and doctoral degree in educational leadership at the University of Phoenix.

Dr. Davis-Kennedy was a Registered Nurse (RN) for four years in the medical surgical trauma and critical care unit. She is currently a certified Family Nurse Practitioner (FNP) that practices primary care medicine, teen and women's health. In order to feed her unfilled appetite for promoting health and wellness she spends her extra time getting others to be physically active and maintain a healthy lifestyle.

She is an advocate for getting and staying physically fit for managing and treating chronic diseases such as high blood pressure, high cholesterol, diabetes, and much more. People join her in her community when she instructs multiple exercise classes and camps in order to build awareness and encourage a healthier lifestyle.

Not only is Dr. Davis-Kennedy a nursing professor, Family Nurse Practitioner, health educator and fitness motivator, but she also shows her passion for health by being a healthy-living motivational speaker and author.

"I aspire to inspire others to transform into their higher capabilities."

–Dr. Katina Davis-Kennedy

Acknowledgments

I want to thank my family and friends for standing behind me and never allowing me to give up on my dreams; especially my mom, mother-in-law, dad, sisters and son. To my very supportive husband, Stephen Kennedy, you have been my rock, my love, and my world.

In addition, I would like to give a personal thanks to my older sister Trenesa Davis for her unwavering support and countless hours of help on this project.

A special thanks to my colleague Shalonna Battle for her expertise and contribution. As well as my publisher, Shanley at Opportune Publishing, for exceptional hard work and dedication to helping me put my idea in stone. To my nephew, Aaron Davis with A Davis Illustration, thank you for designing the book cover.

Last but not least, I would like to thank you for purchasing this book and allowing yourself to become educated on an important topic. You rock!!

Table of contents

Preface

Do you believe you have enough knowledge to have "The Talk" with your child and be 100% accurate when speaking about sex, including Sexually Transmitted Diseases (STDs)?

For those of you who do not, here is a helping hand to get you ready. I have created this guide for parents, students, and those who are seeking to become more knowledgeable about STDs. It is important that before you, as a parent, have the dreaded sex talk with your child, you are aware of the various STDs that can affect the human body. Doing this can allow you to answer any questions your child may have or come up with throughout your big conversation.

When is it a good time to talk to your child about sex?

This is one of the most controversial questions floating around, because you do not want to have the conversation too soon and expose your child to sexual information too early. But you also do not want to let someone else expose them to the wrong information first.

Psychologists believe "The Talk" can start as early as 9 years of age. But definitely should be discussed in their pre-teens (9-12 years old). Unfortunately, sexual activity may occur as early as 9 years old. Once they are nearing or enter middle school, they are exposed to many different sexual advances from others that are usually more experienced and have more information, right or wrong.

There has been a huge epidemic that has recently come to light: Oral sex practices are vastly prevalent in the middle school population. Without being properly prepared your child could become a victim of an STD or an unwanted pregnancy before you have had the opportunity to sit and share your sexual knowledge.

So, ideally you want to beat those outside influences to the punch. *Let's Talk Sex & STDs: A Guide to Prepare Parents for "The Talk"* is here to help you do so when the time is right.

Chapter 1: What is a Sexually Transmitted Disease?

Let's start from the beginning to ensure we are on the same page and all information is consistent and correct.

Sexually Transmitted Diseases are diseases that are transmitted or acquired through sexual contact. They are infectious and can spread through:

- Direct skin-to-skin contact.
- Contact with infected bodily fluids.
- Oral, anal, and vaginal sex.
- Saliva, blood, smoking and the use of drugs/needles.

If there is any type of sexual activity, then there is a risk for a STD!

Sexually Transmitted Diseases are called many different things; don't get confused by different terms because they all can be used interchangeably.

Here is a list of some:

- Sexually Transmitted Disease (STD)

- Sexually Transmitted Infections (STI)

- Venereal Disease (VD)

It is important to highlight that STDs are sexually transmitted, which means they can be passed via sexual activities. For example, if a male does not penetrate the vagina, but does rub or touch the area with his penis, this is a sexual activity. If he were infected with an STD, this would be an example of sexually transmitting. Simply touching genitals increase the risk of contracting genital warts, herpes, and other STDs.

This is also true in regard to oral sex. Just because there is no insertion of the penis into the vagina, absolutely does not mean one cannot contract an STD.

This is the importance of educating yourself and your children on the information regarding Sexually Transmitted Diseases. There are many myths and rumors evolving around sex, but misinformation can lead to death.

Chapter 2: All about STDs

Let's Talk Sex & STDs: A Guide to Prepare Parents for "The Talk" was created to breakdown the myths, tell actual facts and disseminate real information in a way that a parent or child would understand. In this chapter, we will go through an array of STDs; some that can be cured and others that cannot.

You will learn about bacterial, viral, and other STDs along with the signs and symptoms to identify if you suspect a STD has been transmitted. It is important that if you recognize any of these symptoms, you need to seek medical attention immediately. **Do not try to cure yourself at home!**

Taking the appropriate antibiotics and anti-parasitic medications can cure bacterial and parasitic sexually transmitted infections. However, viral STDs, like HIV/AIDS, are not cured but are managed with anti-viral medications. When it comes to viral STDs, once you've contracted them, you own them!! So it is a great time to have "The Talk" to prevent your child from owning such a life-altering gift.

13

Let's Talk Sex & STDs

Chapter 3: Bacterial Sexually Transmitted Diseases

Bacterial sexually transmitted diseases occur when there is a contraction of certain bacterium from another person. This is similar to passing germs to other people and making them sick. These are the STDs that can be cured, luckily.

Chlamydia

Chlamydia is a very common STD, especially among teens. It can be asymptomatic (no symptoms) in females, yet symptomatic in males. If indications are present, they usually show up 7-28 days after having sex with someone who is infected. However, chlamydia can be detected through tests as early as 1-3 weeks after contraction, if tested by urine sample or a genital culture (a sample swab of the discharge from the genitals to detect organisms that are bacterial, viral or fungal infections).

There are several ways one can be infected by chlamydia: Through heterosexual and homosexual intercourse; vaginal, anal and oral sex. If you

15

experience any of the symptoms below, you should seek medical attention immediately.

Symptoms amongst females include:

- An abnormal vaginal discharge.
- A burning sensation or pain when urinating.
- Bleeding in between periods.
- Pain during sex.
- Lower abdominal cramping/pain.

Symptoms amongst males include:

- A watery, white discharge from the penis.
- A burning sensation or pain when urinating.
- Frequent urination.
- Pain and swelling in one or both testicles.

Rectal symptoms in both men and women include:

- Discharge
- Rectal pain
- Bleeding

Remember: Chlamydia can be cured with antibiotics. If untreated, this disease can lead to infertility and other very serious complications. A urine sample or genital culture is used to detect chlamydia.

Chlamydia can affect different parts of the body, as shown below.

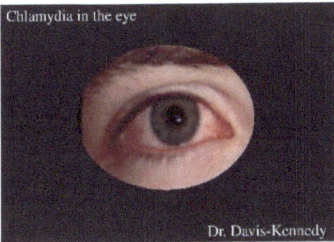
Chlamydia in the eye
Dr. Davis-Kennedy

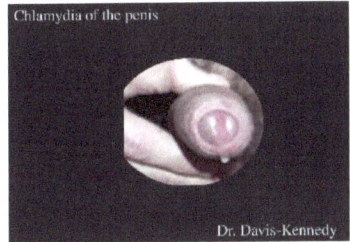
Chlamydia of the penis
Dr. Davis-Kennedy

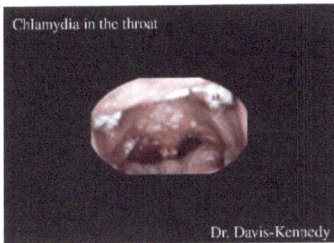
Chlamydia in the throat
Dr. Davis-Kennedy

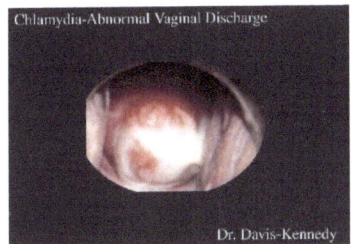
Chlamydia-Abnormal Vaginal Discharge
Dr. Davis-Kennedy

Gonorrhea

Gonorrhea is another common STD, especially among the age group 15-24, according to the Center for Disease Control (CDC). Just like chlamydia, it can be present without symptoms; Asymptomatic in both males and females. But can be detected at least 2-21 days after being infected. However, it is recommended to wait to be tested 2 weeks after possible contraction to ensure accurate results.

Gonorrhea ("the clap" or "the drip") is caused by a bacterium called Neisseria Gonorrhea, which can grow and multiply easily within the body. Common areas include: reproductive tract (cervix, uterus, fallopian tubes and urethra), mouth, throat and anus.

This bacterial infection can be contracted vaginally, anally or orally. If you experience any of the symptoms below, you should seek medical attention immediately.

Gonorrhea indicators in men include:

- A burning sensation or pain when urinating.
- A white, yellow, or green discharge from the penis.
- Pain during sex.
- Abnormal frequency of urination.
- Painful or swollen testicles.

Gonorrhea women indicators include:

- Painful or burning sensation when urinating.
- Green, white or yellow vaginal discharge.
- Lower abdomen pain and cramps.
- Pain during sex.
- Vaginal bleeding between periods.

When a female has gonorrhea symptoms, they are often mild and can be mistaken for a bladder or vaginal infection.

Rectal infections may either have no signs or have indicators in both men and women that may include:

- Discharge
- Anal itching
- Soreness
- Bleeding
- Painful bowel movements

Remember: Gonorrhea can be cured with antibiotics. If untreated, this disease can lead to infertility. A urine sample or genital culture is used to detect gonorrhea. If you experience any of these symptoms, you should seek medical attention immediately.

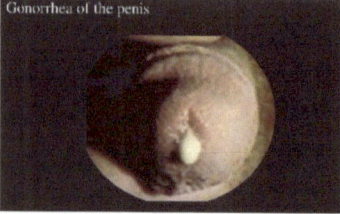

Gonorrhea of the penis

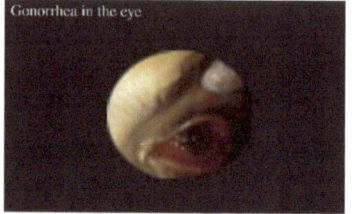

Gonorrhea in the eye

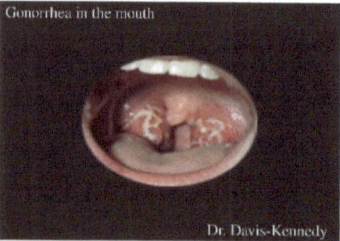

Gonorrhea in the mouth

Dr. Davis-Kennedy

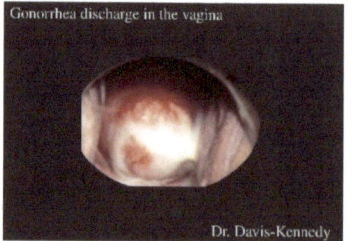

Gonorrhea discharge in the vagina

Dr. Davis-Kennedy

Syphilis

Although Syphilis is not as prevalent today as it was in the 1960s – 1980s many people are still being infected. This highly contagious disease is spread primarily through sexual activity, including oral and anal sex. Other ways it can be passed on is through prolonged kissing, close bodily contact or open sores. Sores can be found on the penis, vagina, and anus. Sometimes found in the rectum, on the lips and in the mouth. Syphilis can also be spread from an infected mother to her unborn baby.

If someone is infected with syphilis, there are several stages they will go through during this infection:

Primary stage: (1-12 weeks after having sex)

- Painless syphilis sore or sores can appear on the mouth or genitals (often confused as an ingrown hair, zipper cut, or harmless bump).

- These sores can last 2-6 weeks.

*Even after sores aren't present anymore, syphilis is still present.

Second Stage: (new symptoms show up as the sores leave)

- A non-itchy rash appearing on hands, soles of feet, all over your body or in just a few places.

21

- You will start experiencing flu-like symptoms: Fever, swollen glands, fatigue, muscle aches, headache and sore throat.

- Weight loss occurs.

*Even after rash and flu-like symptoms go away, syphilis is still present.

Latent Stages: (all previous symptoms have gone away)

- Difficulty coordinating muscle movements.

- Paralysis (unable to move certain parts of your body).

- Numbness, blindness, and dementia (mental disorder).

- Damage to internal organs, which can result in death.

If you experience any of the above symptoms, you should seek medical attention immediately.

Remember: Syphilis can be diagnosed through a blood test. Syphilis is a bacterial infection and can be cured with specific antibiotics. However, treatment will not undo any damage caused by the infection. If you experience any of the symptoms, you should seek medical attention immediately, treatment is time sensitive.

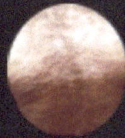

First Stage- Painless Sore
Dr. Davis-Kennedy

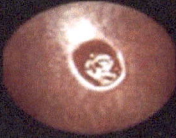

Secondary Stage rash from syphilis on torso.
Dr. Davis-Kennedy

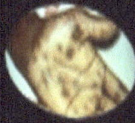

Secondary rash from syphilis on palms of hands
Dr. Davis-Kennedy

Let's Talk Sex & STDs

Chapter 4: Viral Sexually Transmitted Diseases

Viruses passed from person-to-person during sexual activity cause viral STDs. In general these infections involve multiple parts of the body simultaneously. There are several infections in this category, including Genital Herpes, HIV/AIDS, Hepatitis B, Hepatitis C and HPV. These are the most serious of all infections to get; they cannot be cured, but there are many types of treatments so that one can continue to live.

Hepatitis B

The word hepatitis means "inflammation of the liver". Hepatitis B is a virus that can cause scarring of the liver, liver failure, and liver diseases such as cirrhosis and liver cancer.

Hepatitis B is usually transmitted through sex, but can be caused by other things as well; i.e. toxins, certain drugs, some diseases, heavy alcohol use and bacterial and viral infections. In the U.S. among adults Hepatitis B is usually spread through sexual contact and accounts for nearly two-thirds of acute Hepatitis B cases.

Believe it or not, Hepatitis B can be up to 100 times more infectious than HIV. It can be contracted through oral sex with an infected person, male or female.

Hepatitis B can also be spread by:

- Coming in contact with infected blood.
- Sharing needles, razors or toothbrushes with an infected person.
- Childbirth from an infected mother to her baby.

Symptoms for Hepatitis B show up 1-9 months after transmission from someone who has Hepatitis B, and are mild or nonexistent.

Women and men with symptoms may notice the following:

- Flu-like symptoms that don't go away.
- Fatigue Jaundice (yellow skin)
- Joint Pain
- Fever
- Loss of appetite
- Nausea
- Vomiting
- Dark urine
- Light-colored bowel movements.

Remember: Hepatitis B is a viral infection and there is no cure for it. However, there is a vaccine available to protect you from contracting this virus. If you feel you may have come in contact with someone with this infection, a simple blood test is used to detect this virus for diagnosis. If left untreated for a time, it can result in needing a liver transplant, or death.

Hepatitis C

Hepatitis C is very similar to Hepatitis B; you can be infected the same ways:

- From toxins, certain drugs, some diseases and heavy alcohol use.
- Bacterial and viral infections, infected blood, sharing needles, razors and toothbrushes.
- Sexual transmission and childbirth.

In addition, Hepatitis C can be transmitted in other ways, such as getting a tattoo.

Many people have no symptoms or mild symptoms. Symptoms usually appear 6-7 weeks after exposure to Hepatitis C. However, this can range from 2 weeks to 6 months in certain cases.

Women and men with symptoms may notice the following:

- Flu-like symptoms that don't go away.
- Fatigue
- Jaundice (yellow skin)
- Joint Pain
- Fever
- Loss of appetite
- Nausea
- Vomiting
- Dark urine
- Light-colored bowel movements.

Remember: There is no cure for the Hepatitis C virus. However, medications are used to manage this disease. But no cure has been found just yet. If you suspect you may have Hepatitis C, seek medical attention immediately to get a blood test for possible diagnosis. If left untreated, it can result in needing a liver transplant, or death.

Genital Herpes

Genital herpes is a very common Sexually Transmitted Disease caused by the contraction of two viruses: Herpes simplex type 1 and Herpes simplex type 2.

In the United States, about one out of every six people aged 14 to 49 years have genital herpes. You can get herpes by having vaginal, anal or oral sex, as well as genital-to-genital contact with someone who has this viral disease.

The virus is actually carried in the fluid found within the herpes sores; contact with this fluid will cause infection. Even if there are no visible sores, contact with an infected person can cause transmission of genital herpes.

Symptoms can show up 1-30 days or later after having sex. Most people have no symptoms or mild ones.

Women and men with symptoms may notice the following:

- Flu-like feelings (fever, body aches, or swollen glands).

- Small, painful blisters on the genitals, rectum or mouth (often mistaken as a painful pimple or ingrown hair).
- Itching or burning before blisters appear.
- Blister may go away, but you still have herpes; blisters can come back.

Remember: This is a viral infection that can be spread very easily. Even if a person is a virgin, they may contract genital herpes if they come in contact with infected genitals. Unfortunately, condoms do not protect against genital herpes because it is spread through skin-to-skin contact. There is no cure for Herpes, but medications can be used to stop or manage outbreaks. You can request a HSV-1 and HSV-2 blood test to confirm if this virus is present.

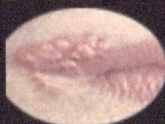

Herpes of the vagina

Dr. Davis-Kennedy

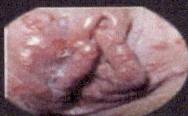

Herpes of the mouth

Dr. Davis-Kennedy

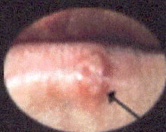

Herpes of the mouth

Dr. Davis-Kennedy

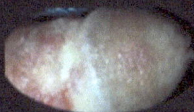

Herpes of the penis

Dr. Davis-Kennedy

HIV/AIDS

The Human Immunodeficiency Virus (HIV) is the immune system attacker that can lead to Development of Acquired Immunodeficiency Syndrome (AIDS). Unlike other infections, the human body cannot get rid of HIV/AIDS. Unfortunately, once you have HIV you have it forever. There is only one-way to know if you are infected; you must test by blood or oral fluid analysis.

HIV is often considered the most serious and dangerous STD existing. This is a virus that you cannot see and symptoms aren't always reliable. Many people who are infected with HIV may not have any symptoms for 10 years or more.

It can be transmitted through oral sex with someone, heterosexual or homosexual, that is infected. HIV can also be spread through infected blood, sharing of needles, syringes, or other drug-injection equipment.

Other ways HIV can be contracted:

- Sharing razors or toothbrushes with an infected person.

- Through breast milk and direct contact with the blood or open sores of an infected person.

- Through childbirth (spread from an infected mother to her baby during birth)

*Medications are commonly used to stop the transmission to the baby.

HIV is a sexually transmitted disease that can be dormant and have an incubation period for an extended amount of time. This means that it can go undetected, even if a person is, in fact, infected.

HID/AIDS Indicators:

- Flu-like symptoms (the worst flu ever usually 2 to 4 weeks after exposure).
- Fever
- Enlarged lymph nodes.
- Unexplained weight loss and/or fatigue.
- Diarrhea
- White spots in mouth.
- Yeast infection in women that don't go away.
- Sore throat
- Rash

These symptoms can last anywhere from a few days to several weeks. Even if HIV cannot be detected at the time, it is highly infectious and can be spread to others.

Types of Tests to detect HIV/AIDS:

Antibody tests ("Rapid" tests) — Gives a result based on antibodies to HIV, not the virus itself. It can properly start detection 2-8 weeks after infection exposure; most people will have enough antibodies to test precisely. Twelve weeks after initial infection, about 97% of people will have enough antibodies to test accurately.

Antigen tests (RNA tests) — Show a result based on the presence of the virus within the body. These tests are more expensive than antibody tests, so are not offered in as many places. A 1-3 week after infection exposure is usually enough time for a proper result using this RNA tests.

Remember: There is no cure for HIV but there are many different treatment options to manage the virus. This is no longer the disease that you have to die from. If you are not treated and do not take care of your body, it will eventually turn into AIDS, which is a lot more severe.

You must get tested before a new partner and after you have changed partners. If you have unprotected sex, it is recommended you get blood tested two weeks, three months, six months, and a year after the unprotected sexual encounter.

Human Papillomavirus (HPV)

HPV is the absolute most common sexually transmitted infection (STI) according to the CDC. Nearly all sexually active men and women get it at some point in their lives. About 79 million Americans are currently infected and nearly 14 million new people become infected each year.

You can get HPV by having vaginal, anal or oral sex, as well as genital touching (skin-to-skin contact) with someone who has the disease. Symptoms can show up weeks, months, or years after contact with HPV. Many people have no symptoms at all ever in life.

There are many different types of HPV; women and men can get different types. Different types cause different symptoms such as:

Genital Warts - Single or group of bumpy warts on the genitals. Genital Warts can be small or large, raised or flat, or shaped like a cauliflower. They cause itching or burning around the sex organs. The warts may go away, but they can return at any time because the virus stays in the body forever.

Cancer - Cell changes to cancerous within the cervix, vulva, vagina, penis, anus, and throat.

This virus is not easily avoided; virgins can get HPV/Genital Warts and condoms do not protect against Genital Warts, being that it is spread through skin-to-skin contact.

Although there is no cure for HPV, there is a vaccine called Gardasil that is safe and effective. The Gardasil vaccine is approved for both males and females between the ages of 9-26, and is recommended before the first time having sexual activity or intercourse. This vaccine protects from genital warts and high-risk cancer causing HPV strands.

Remember: There is no blood test at this time to check for HPV. It cannot be detected in men, but women can request a pap smear to check for HPV. Pap smears are recommended for women between the ages of 21 and 65 years old and can prevent the progression cervical cancer.

Let's Talk Sex & STDs

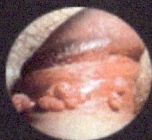
HPV of the penis
Dr. Davis-Kennedy

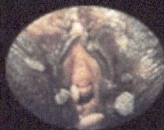
HPV of the vagina
Dr. Davis-Kennedy

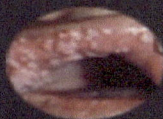
HPV of mouth
Dr. Davis-Kennedy

Chapter 5: Other STD's

A lot of the STDs mentioned in previous chapters are amongst the most common of them all. Believe it or not, there are even more sexually transmitted diseases. There is not a lot of mention of Parasitic STDs, but they do exist. It is important that when educating someone on a topic, you give him or her the full scope. So, next we are going to discuss less known STDs, some parasitic and more bacterial and viral infections as well.

Trichomoniasis (Trich)

Trichomoniasis is a sexually transmitted disease that is caused by infection of a protozoan parasite called Trichomonas Vaginalis. It is considered to be the most common curable STD. In the United States, an estimated 3.7 million people have the infection, but only about 30% develop any symptoms of Trichomoniasis, according to the CDC.

Although symptoms vary, most people who have the parasite cannot tell they are infected at all. It is transferred during vaginal sex. In women, the most commonly infected part of the body is the lower genital tract:

In women: vulva, vagina, or urethra.

In men: inside of the penis (urethra).

If symptoms ever show up, it's usually 5-28 days after having sex with an infected person.

Men with symptoms may have:

- A burning sensation or pain when urinating.
- A watery white drip from penis.
- Frequent urination.

Women with symptoms may have:

- Itching, burning, or irritation in the vagina.
- Fishy or musky odor from the vagina.
- Yellow, greenish, or gray vaginal discharge.
- Vaginal bleeding between periods.

Remember: Trich can be cured with antibiotics. The diagnosis comes from a genital culture in both men and women. Trich is also seen in homosexual women and those who share sex toys without cleaning it properly first.

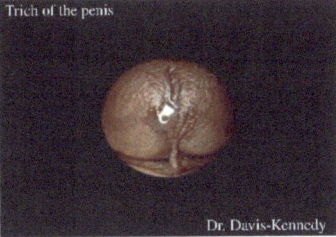

Trich of the penis
Dr. Davis-Kennedy

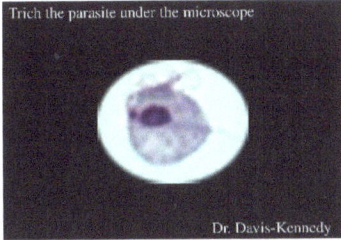

Trich the parasite under the microscope
Dr. Davis-Kennedy

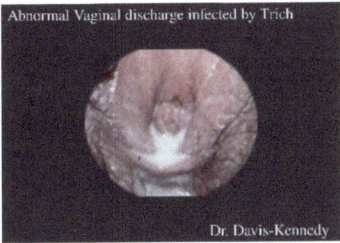

Abnormal Vaginal discharge infected by Trich
Dr. Davis-Kennedy

Chancroid

Chancroid is a sexually transmitted genital ulcer disease caused by the bacterium Haemophilus Ducreyi. Although not as common in the United States, it is a relatively common disease in the developing world. Chancroid is transmitted through vaginal and anal sex. Symptoms usually show up 1 week after having sex.

Symptoms may include:

- One or more painful genital ulcer.
- Lymph node enlargement where the Chancroid is located.

Remember: A genital culture is used to detect Chancroid and it can be cured with antibiotics. It's common in some regions of Africa and in the Caribbean.

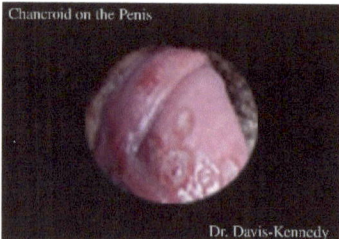

Chancroid on the Penis

Dr. Davis-Kennedy

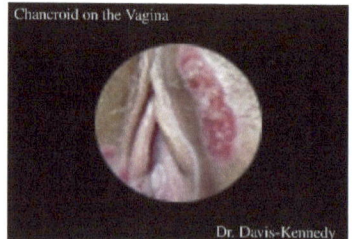

Chancroid on the Vagina

Dr. Davis-Kennedy

Lymphogranuloma Venereum (LGV)

LGV is a sexually transmitted disease or infection involving the lymph glands in the genital area. It is caused by a specific strain of Chlamydia; which comes from bacteria. Lymphogranuloma Venereum is transmitted via vaginal and anal sex.

The occurrence of LGV is highest among sexually active people in tropical or subtropical environments. It has also occurred in some areas of the southern United States.

Symptoms show up 3-30 days after having sex with an infected person.

Symptoms may include:

- Painless small sore on the penis or vagina.
- Enlarged genital lymph nodes.
- Infection can spread to the lymph node in the groin area if not treated.

Remember: A genital culture and blood test is used to detect this disease, and antibiotics cure it. LGV is common in tropical or subtropical climates.

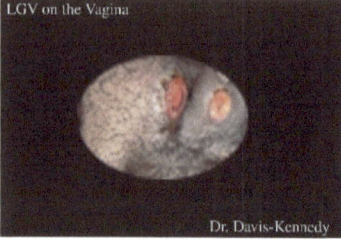

LGV on the Vagina

Dr. Davis-Kennedy

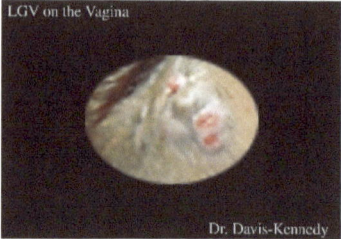

LGV on the Vagina

Dr. Davis-Kennedy

Pediculosis Pubis

Pediculosis Pubis, also known as Pubic Lice or Crabs, are small parasitic bugs that reside in the pubic area. Pubic lice are parasitic insects found primarily in the pubic or genital area of humans and feed off blood. Pubic lice infestation is found worldwide and occurs in all races, ethnic groups, and levels of society.

Pubic lice are transmitted through bed sheets, sexual contact, vaginal and anal sex, and genital rubbing.

Symptoms show up immediately or up to 1 day after being infected.

Symptoms may include:

- Itching in the genital area.
- Visible nits (lice/bug eggs).
- Visible crawling lice/bugs.

Remember: Pubic Lice/Crabs can be cured with anti-parasitic medication. It is less commonly found in eyebrows, eyelashes, beard, mustache, armpit, perianal area, groin, trunk, and scalp. A healthcare provider seeing the bugs with or without a microscope detects this parasitic disease.

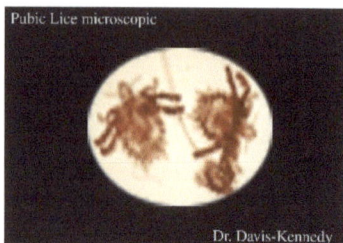

Pubic Lice microscopic

Dr. Davis-Kennedy

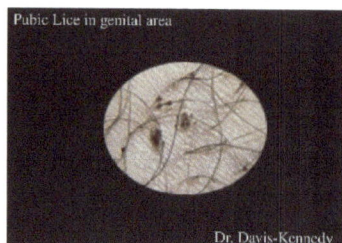

Pubic Lice in genital area

Dr. Davis-Kennedy

Scabies

Human scabies is caused by an infestation of the skin by the human itch mite (Sarcoptes scabiei var. hominis). These very small parasitic bugs burrow into the upper layer of the skin where it lives and lays its eggs.

Scabies are spread by direct, prolonged, skin-to-skin contact with a person who is infected. Sexual activities are a great way to become inhabited by these mites.

For first time scabies, symptoms may take as long as 4-6 weeks to show up. It is imperative to remember that an infected person can spread scabies at all times, even if symptoms are not present. In a person who has had scabies before, symptoms usually appear much sooner; usually 1-4 days after re-exposure.

Symptoms may include:

- Intense itching in these areas: the wrist, elbow, armpit, between fingers, nipple, penis, waist, belt-line, and buttocks.
- Pimple-like skin rash.

Remember: The healthcare provider seeing the bugs, with or without a microscope, detects this parasitic disease. If detected, Scabies can be cured with anti-parasitic medication.

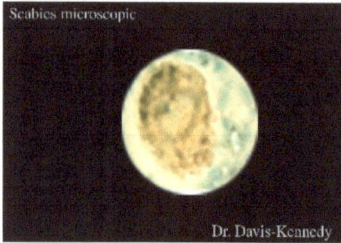

Scabies microscopic

Dr. Davis-Kennedy

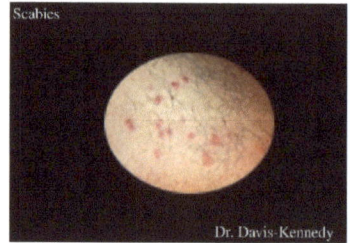

Scabies

Dr. Davis-Kennedy

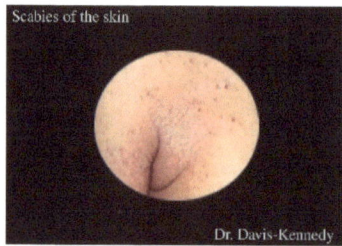

Scabies of the skin

Dr. Davis-Kennedy

Molluscum

Molluscum Contagiosum is an infection caused by a poxvirus: Molluscum Contagiosum. The visual effect is usually a benign, mild skin disease characterized by lesions or growths on the body. Molluscum may occur anywhere on the body; i.e. the face, neck, arms, legs, abdomen, and genital area, all at once or region based. The lesions are rarely found on the palms of the hands or the soles of the feet, so if you notice lesions in these areas, it may be something else.

Molluscum usually spreads by direct skin-to-skin contact with an infected person. This can be transmitted when having sexual intercourse with a person who is infected thus making it a sexually transmitted disease.

Symptoms can appear 2-12 weeks after exposure; however it can take years for it to appear to the eye.

Symptoms may include:

- Lesion/bump that is small, raised, and usually white, pink, or flesh-colored with a dimple or pit in the center.
- Pearly-appearing bump that is smooth and firm.
- Bumps/lesions that may be itchy, sore, red, and/or swollen.

Remember: This disease is detected by inspection by your healthcare provider. There are medications available that you can take orally or apply directly to the skin. However, your healthcare provider may burn or freeze the bumps away. Within 6-12 months, Molluscum Contagiosum typically resolves without scarring but can take as long as 4 years to do so. Since the virus lives only on the top layer of skin, once the lesions are gone the virus is gone and you cannot spread it to others.

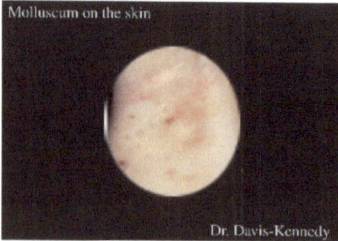

Molluscum on the skin
Dr. Davis-Kennedy

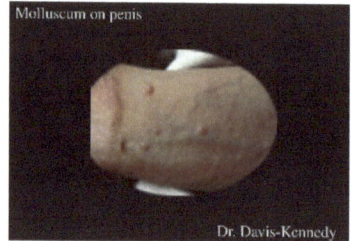

Molluscum on penis
Dr. Davis-Kennedy

Chapter 6: Parental Do's and Don'ts

As a parent, it may be difficult to discuss sex with your child; especially if they are still as young as 9 years old. However, the reality is they will have sex! Hopefully, later than sooner, but whenever that time comes we can make sure they are properly prepared.

Before you actually have "The Talk," you may want to consider a few things. The aforementioned chapters have equipped you with the information to share, but now you have to actually disseminate said information properly so that it does not intimidate your child or create an intense fear. Ideally, you want to have a comfortable, inviting and calm environment so that your child knows sex is normal and it's important to have an open discussion about it.

Here is some recommended advice for "The Talk":

- It is important to be knowledgeable about sex yourself to make sure proper information is given and you are comfortable passing that information to your child.

- Study all the information in chapters 1 – 5 to make sure you know the names of the STDs, how to contract them and the symptoms for each.

- Be open-minded. This may or may not be the first time your child has heard about sex. So, be open to what they already know or want to know. This will make way for open and honest dialogue.

- Assess what your child already knows. Many adolescents talk about sex, but their knowledge base is usually full of rumors, myths and a little of the actual truth. This will allow you to do away with the false information and replace it with facts.

- Talk with your child, not at your child. Many parents go into lecture mode when having discussions. But remember the idea is to keep it a conversation so she/he will feel comfortable enough to ask questions and be open with you.

- If by chance your teen admits to having sexual intercourse or some sort of sexual activity, do not react in a negative manner. This will cause your child not to talk to you again about sexual issues. Just take a deep breath and be understanding so you both can move forward.

- Be sympathetic. Remember you have been in those scary shoes as well. The student is usually always just as scared as the teacher. Say some of the things you wished your parent would have said to you.
- Continuously promote being approachable. This will make room for future conversations, which could prevent unwanted pregnancies, STDs or premature sexual encounters.
- It is important that you communicate your family values, which serves as a reminder of its significant that you keep them safe, equip them with proper tools and whatever else you want them to know about sex or abstinence.
- If your child is already sexually active, or plans to become active soon, schedule a doctor's appointment to go over contraceptives and health screenings.

Let's Talk Sex & STDs

Chapter 7: Advice to Include

Sex is a risky activity people engage in, it shouldn't be looked at as just fun or something that people just do.

After you have your list of everything you want to include in "The Talk," be sure to add your advice as a parent. Some things to include can be:

- Talk to your parent before engaging in sexual activities.
- See a doctor before having sex.
- Start birth control before you have sex.
- Make sure you understand what STDs are and what they can do to a person before you engage in any sexual activities.
- Get tested for STDs before you decide to have sex; your partner as well.
- Know your future sexual partner very well, and enter a monogamous relationship.
- Know your partner sexual history. Ask if they have ever been tested and have ever had an STD.
- Examine your partner thoroughly before sexual activity.

- Learn how to use both male and female condoms and other contraceptives.
- If engaging in oral sex, use Dental Dam.
- Don't ask your friends about sex, because they will have the wrong information.
- Absolutely do not have unprotected sex.
- Do not have sex with people you do not know well.

Chapter 8: Wrap Up

In a nutshell...How can one prevent themselves from getting STDs?

It is vital to remind your child to protect themselves. Either with condoms or abstain from engaging in sex. Unfortunately, condoms do not always prevent one from getting an STD. Some sexually transmitted infections can spread via the skin not covered by the condom. Abstinence is the best way not to get a STD. But the reality is people will have sex.

As you have read, there are many STDs that are bacterial, viral, and parasitic. If you get a bacteria or parasitic STD you have been given a second chance because there is a cure. However, if you catch a viral STD this cannot be cured, unfortunately. Once you got it, you own it!

Sexually transmitted diseases are transmitted via skin-to-skin contact and through vaginal, oral, and anal sex. Virgins can get STDs too with some sexual activities like touching genitals with another person that has a sexually transmitted disease.

Remember, it should be the No.1 priority that if your child does, or eventually will, have sex that they use male or female condoms properly every time they have sex. If they have a latex allergy, no worries!! There are condoms made out of Polyurethane such as Trojan Supra or Durex Avanti that can be used.

For oral sex, be sure to explain the importance of the use of a Dental Dam. Promote being in a long-term mutually monogamous relationship with a partner who has been tested and has negative STD test results. This will also decrease risks of getting a STD.

When a person engages in risky sexual activities, there are consequences. It is great to be that influencer of making responsible decisions and being knowledgeable about sex.

You are now ready for "The Talk."

Glossary

Anal Sex- The insertion and thrusting of an erect penis into an anus for sexual pleasure.

Anti-parasitic Medications- Medications that are indicated for the treatment of parasitic diseases.

Anti-viral Medications- Medications that are indicated for the treatment of viral diseases.

Antibiotics- A type of antimicrobial used in the treatment and prevention of bacterial infections. They may either kill or inhibit the growth of bacteria.

Antibody/Antigen Test- Tests done to find certain antibodies that attack red blood cells.

Asymptomatic- Producing or showing no symptoms.

Bacterial Infection- An infection caused by bacteria.

Bacterium- A microscopic living organism, usually one-celled, that can be found everywhere.

Bodily Fluids- Liquids originating from inside the bodies of living humans.

Cancer- The disease caused by an uncontrolled division of abnormal cells in a part of the body.

Chancroid- A venereal infection causing ulceration of the lymph nodes in the groin.

Chlamydia- A common sexually transmitted infection caused by a very small bacterium.

Contraceptives- A device or drug used in order to prevent pregnancy.

Crabs- (Slang for Pubic Lice) Parasitic insects that can infest in the genital area.

Dental Dam- A thin sheet of latex used as a prophylactic device during oral sex.

Diagnosis- The identification of the nature of an illness or other problem by examination of the symptoms.

Discharge- A secretion coming from the vagina or penis.

Fungal Infection- An infection caused by Fungus.

Genital Culture- A swab analysis of the genitals for the identification of pathogen, whether bacterial, viral, or fungal.

Genital Warts- A small growth occurring in the anal or genital areas caused by Human Papillomavirus (HPV) and is spread by sexual contact.

Genitals- External reproductive organs.

Gonorrhea- A sexually transmitted disease involving inflammatory discharge from the urethra or vagina.

Haemophilus Ducreyi- A fastidious gram-negative coccobacillus causing the sexually transmitted disease chancroid.

Hepatitis B- A severe form of viral hepatitis transmitted in infected blood, causing fever, debility, and jaundice.

Hepatitis C- Inflammation of the liver caused by a severe form of viral hepatitis transmitted through infected blood.

Herpes- A virus causing contagious sores, most often around the mouth or on the genitals.

Heterosexual- Sexually attracted to people of the opposite sex.

HIV/AIDS- Human Immunodeficiency Virus is a virus that attacks the immune system, the body's natural defense system. This causes Acquired Immunodeficiency Syndrome, a chronic, potentially life-threatening condition.

Homosexual- Sexually attracted to people of one's own sex.

HPV- Human papillomavirus, a virus with subtypes that cause diseases in humans ranging from common warts to cervical cancer.

HSV 1 and HSV2 blood test- Testing is performed to identify an acute herpes infection or to detect herpes antibodies.

Infertility- The inability to achieve pregnancy.

Inflammation- A localized physical condition in which part of the body becomes reddened, swollen, hot, and often painful, especially as a reaction to injury or infection.

Intercourse- The act of having sex.

Lymphogranuloma Venereum- A contagious venereal disease caused by various strains of a chlamydia.

Molluscum Contagiosum- A chronic viral disorder of the skin characterized by groups of small, smooth, painless pinkish nodules.

Neisseria Gonorrhea- Type of diplococci bacteria responsible for the sexually transmitted infection gonorrhea.

Oral Sex- The insertion and thrusting of an erect penis or vagina into the mouth for sexual pleasure.

Pap Smear- A procedure to test for cervical cancer in women.

Parasitic Infection- An infectious disease caused or transmitted by a parasite.

Pediculosis Pubis - ("Crabs" or "Pubic Lice") A disease caused by the pubic lice, Pthirus pubis, a parasitic insect that infest human pubic hair.

Protozoan Parasite- A one-celled organism (called protists) that live as a parasite.

Pubic Lice- Slang for Crabs or Public Lice, parasitic insects that can infest in the genital area.

Reproductive Tract- A part of the reproductive system.

Sarcoptes Scabiei Var. Hominis- Little mites that cause scabies, they burrow into the upper layer of the skin to live and lay its eggs.

Scabies- A contagious skin disease marked by itching and small raised red spots, caused by the itch mite (Sarcoptes Scabiei Var. Hominis).

Sexual Activities- Associated with sexual intercourse, but not only the act itself.

Sexually Transmitted Disease (STD)- Any of various diseases or infections that are usually transmitted by direct sexual contact and that include some that may be contracted by other than sexual means.

Sexually Transmitted Infections (STI)- Any of various diseases or infections that are usually transmitted by direct sexual contact and that include some that may be contracted by other than sexual means.

Skin-to-skin contact- Touching another person's skin with any part of your skin.

Trichomonas Vaginalis- An anaerobic flagellated protozoan parasite and the causative agent of **trichomoniasis**.

Trichomoniasis- An infection caused by parasitic trichomonads, chiefly affecting the urinary tract, vagina, or digestive system.

Unprotected Sex- An act of sexual intercourse performed without the use of a condom.

Urethra- The duct by which urine is conveyed out of the body from the bladder.

Vaginal Sex- The insertion and thrusting of an erect penis into a vagina for sexual pleasure.

Venereal Disease (VD)- A disease typically contracted by sexual contact with a person already infected; a sexually transmitted disease.

Viral Infection- A disease that can be caused by different kinds of viruses.

Viruses- An infective agent that typically consists of a nucleic acid molecule in a protein coat, is too small to be seen by light microscopy, and is able to multiply only within the living cells of a host.

References

Center for Disease Control. (2014). Chlamydia CDC fact sheet. Retrieved from http://www.cdc.gov/std/chlamydia/stdfact-chlamydia.htm

Center for Disease Control. (2014). Gonorrhea CDC fact sheet. Retrieved from http://www.cdc.gov/std/chlamydia/stdfact-gonorrhea.htm

Center for Disease Control. (2014). Hepatitis B FAQs for the public. Retrieved from http://www.cdc.gov/hepatitis/hbv/bfaq.htm

Center for Disease Control. (2014). Hepatitis C FAQs for the public. Retrieved from http://www.cdc.gov/hepatitis/hcv/cfaq.htm

Center for Disease Control. (2014). Genital Herpes CDC fact sheet. Retrieved from http://www.cdc.gov/std/herpes/stdfact-herpes.htm

Center for Disease Control. (2015). Genital HPV infection fact sheet. Retrieved from http://www.cdc.gov/std/hpv/stdfact-hpv.htm

Center for Disease Control. (2014). Syphilis CDC fact sheet. Retrieved from http://www.cdc.gov/std/syphilis/stdfact-syphilis.htm

Center for Disease Control. (2015). About HIV/AIDS. Retrieved from http://www.cdc.gov/hiv/basics/whatIshiv.html

San Franscisco AIDS Foundation. (2015). HIV test window periods. Retrieved from http://www.sfaf.org/hiv-info/testing/hiv-test-window-periods.html

Center for Disease Control. (2015). Trichomonas CDC fact sheet. Retrieved from http://www.cdc.gov/std/trichomonas/stdfact-trichomoniasis.htm

Center for Disease Control. (2015). Chancroid. Retrieved from http://www.cdc.gov/std/tg2015/chancroid.htm

Center for Disease Control. (2015). Lymphogranuloma Venereum. Retrieved from http://www.cdc.gov/std/tg2015/lgv.htm

Center for Disease Control. (2014). Pubic Lice. Retrieved from http://www.cdc.gov/parasites/lice/pubic/

Center for Disease Control. (2014). Scabies. Retrieved from http://www.cdc.gov/parasites/scabies/

Center for Disease Control. (2015). Molluscum Contagiosum. Retrieved from http://www.cdc.gov/poxvirus/molluscum-contagiosum/